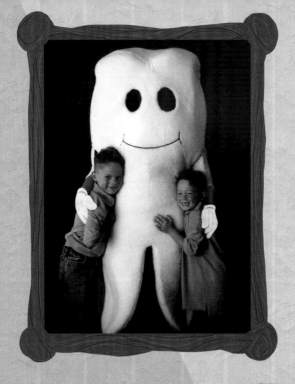

For all you parents who have gone through times in your children's lives where they just flat out refused to brush their teeth, please rest assured that you are not alone! My boys both went through such a phase, despite me being a dentist. I created Mighty Molarman to be the dental health superhero to come to the rescue and save the day!

My hope is that Mighty Molarman & Friends will bring education, resources, and smiles to families around the world.

The Molar, the Merrier!

Dr. John Bond

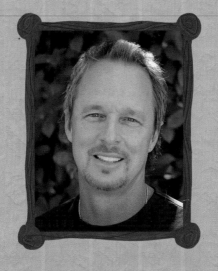

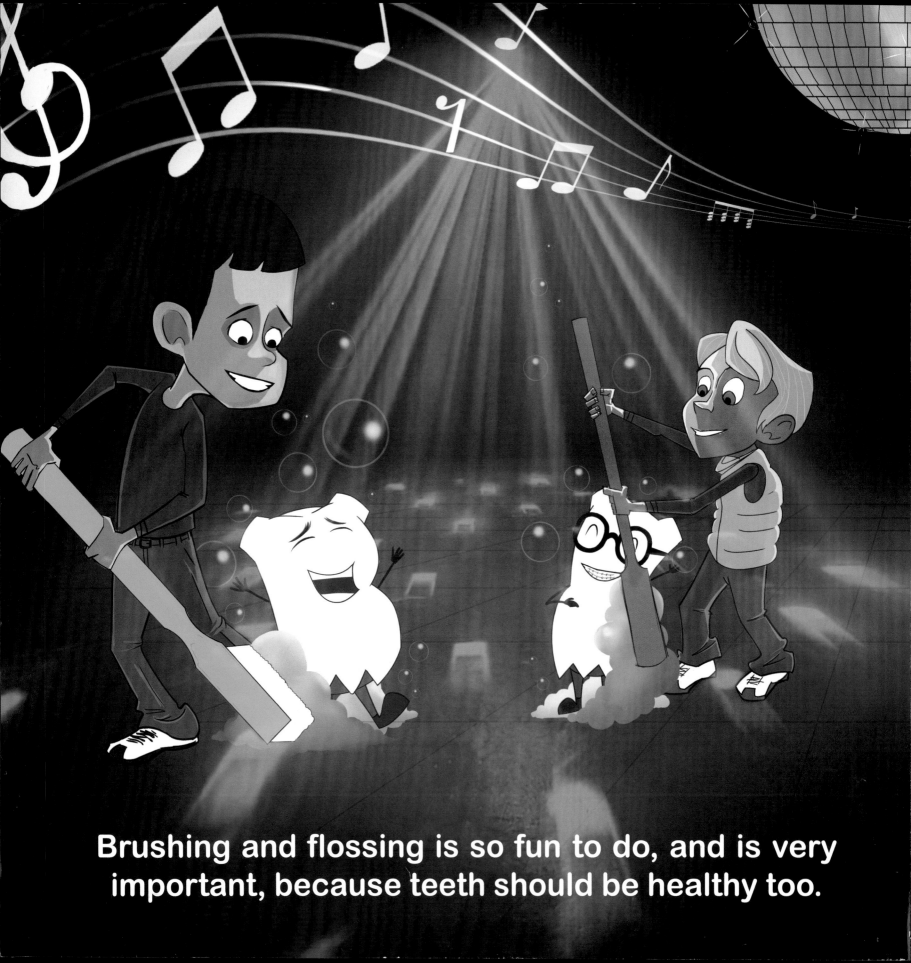

Brushing and flossing is so fun to do, and is very important, because teeth should be healthy too.

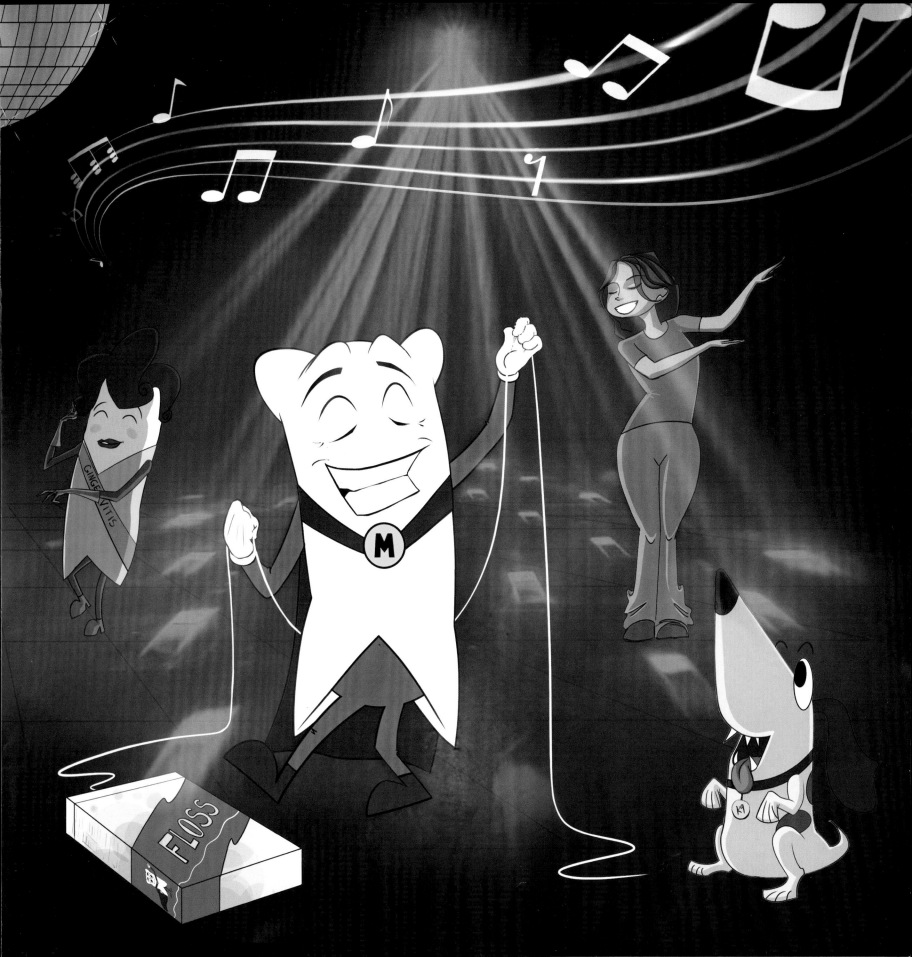

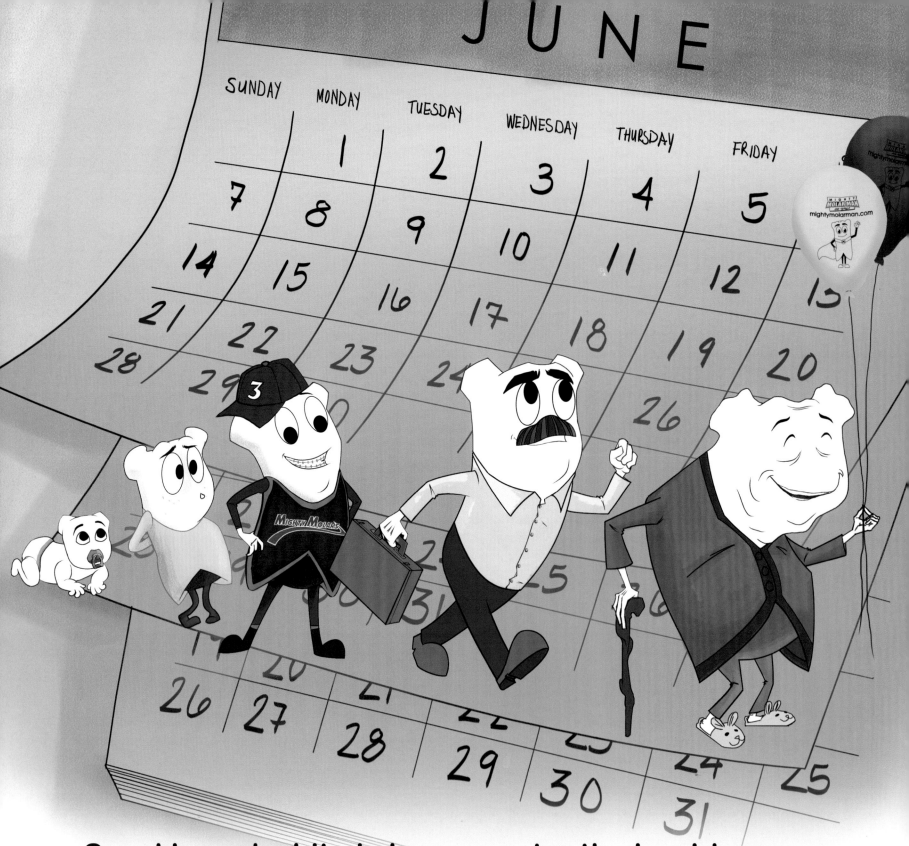

**Sparkly and white is how your teeth should appear,
so clean them really well, year after year.**

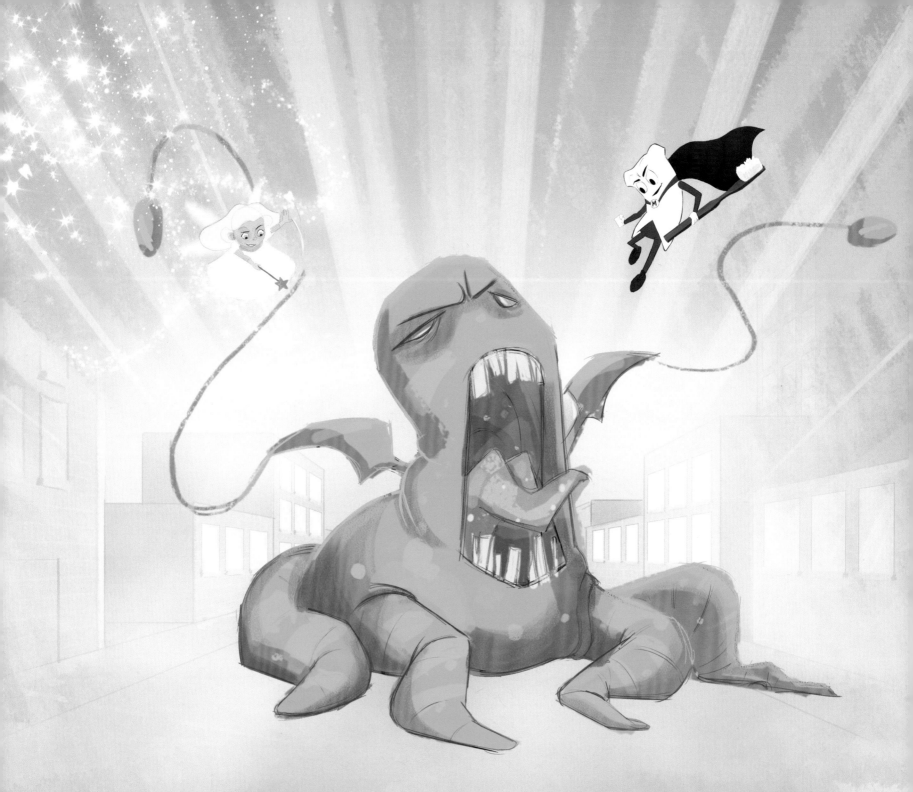

The "Molar in the Mirror", well just who is this fellow?
Why, he is the Tooth Fairy's best friend, who will
help you fight off the yellow.

You see, the Tooth Fairy needs help from time to time.
She found a pearly white partner, who really knows
how to shine.

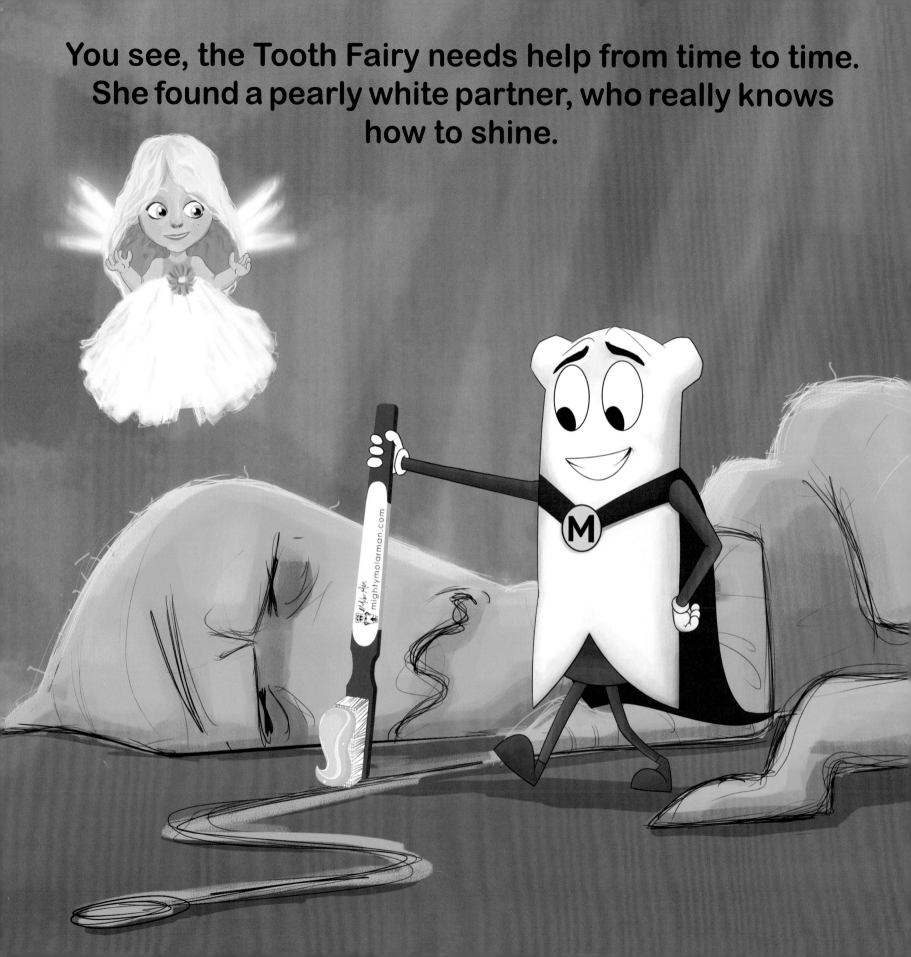

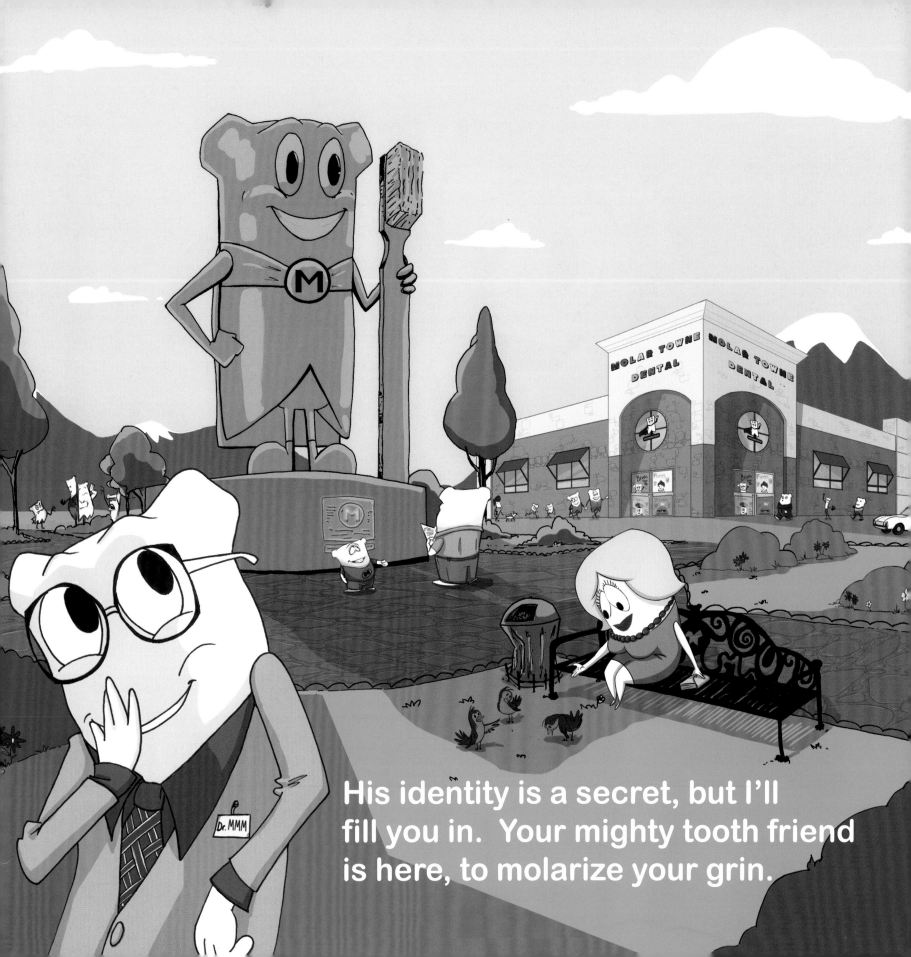

His identity is a secret, but I'll fill you in. Your mighty tooth friend is here, to molarize your grin.

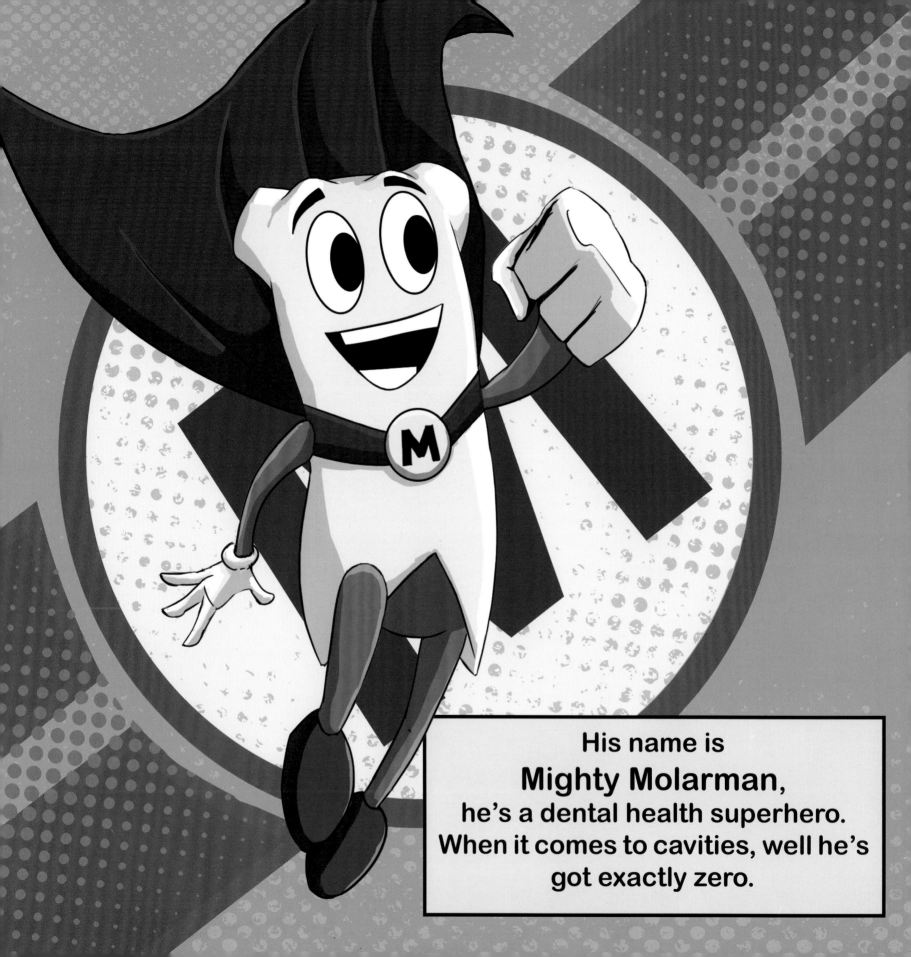

His name is
Mighty Molarman,
he's a dental health superhero.
When it comes to cavities, well he's
got exactly zero.

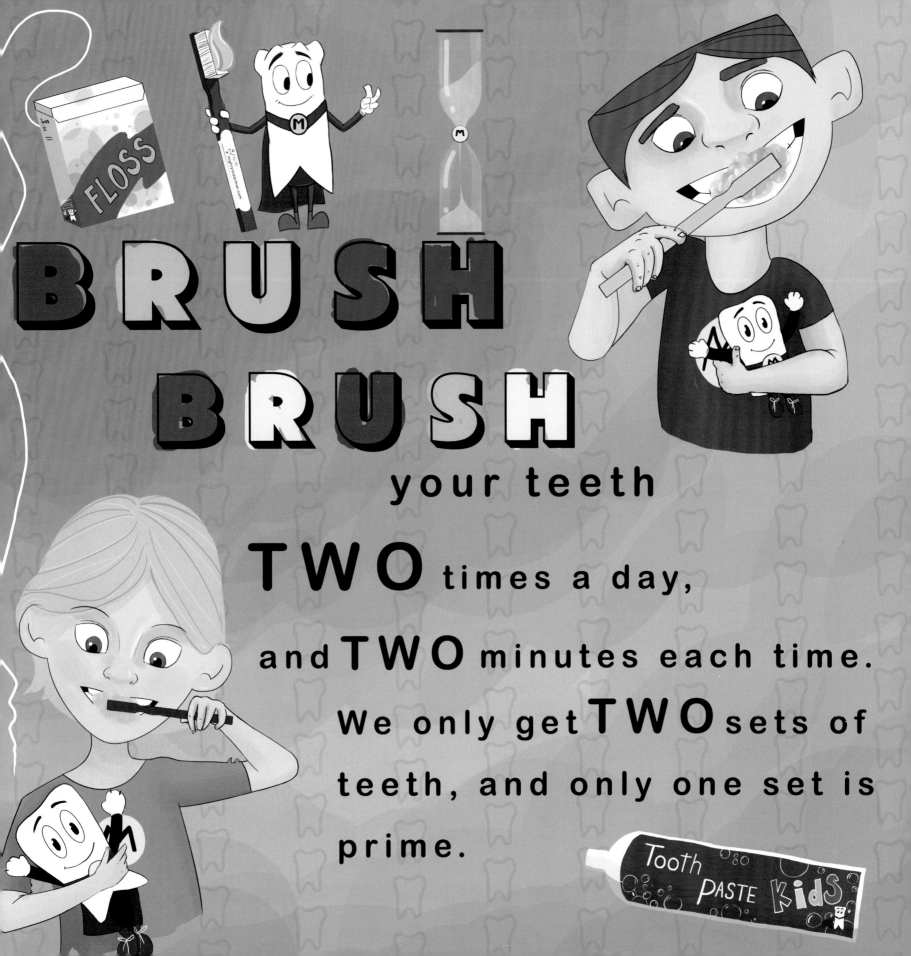

BRUSH BRUSH your teeth **TWO** times a day, and **TWO** minutes each time. We only get **TWO** sets of teeth, and only one set is prime.

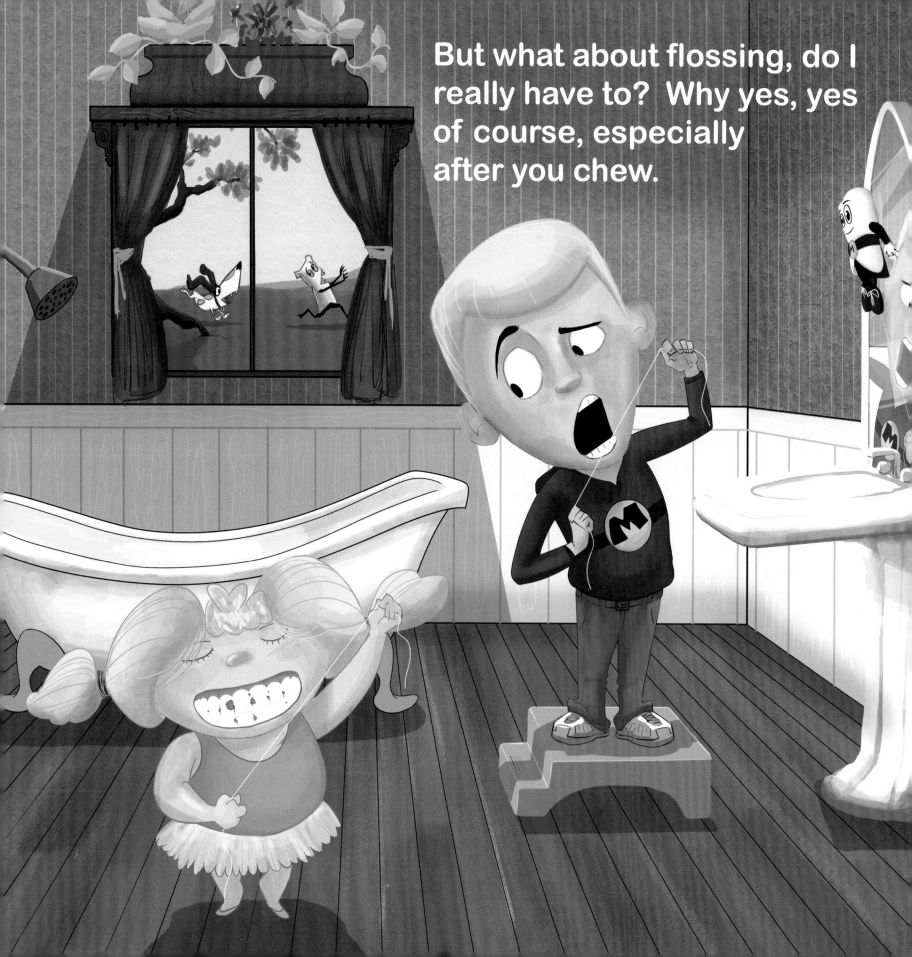

But what about flossing, do I really have to? Why yes, yes of course, especially after you chew.

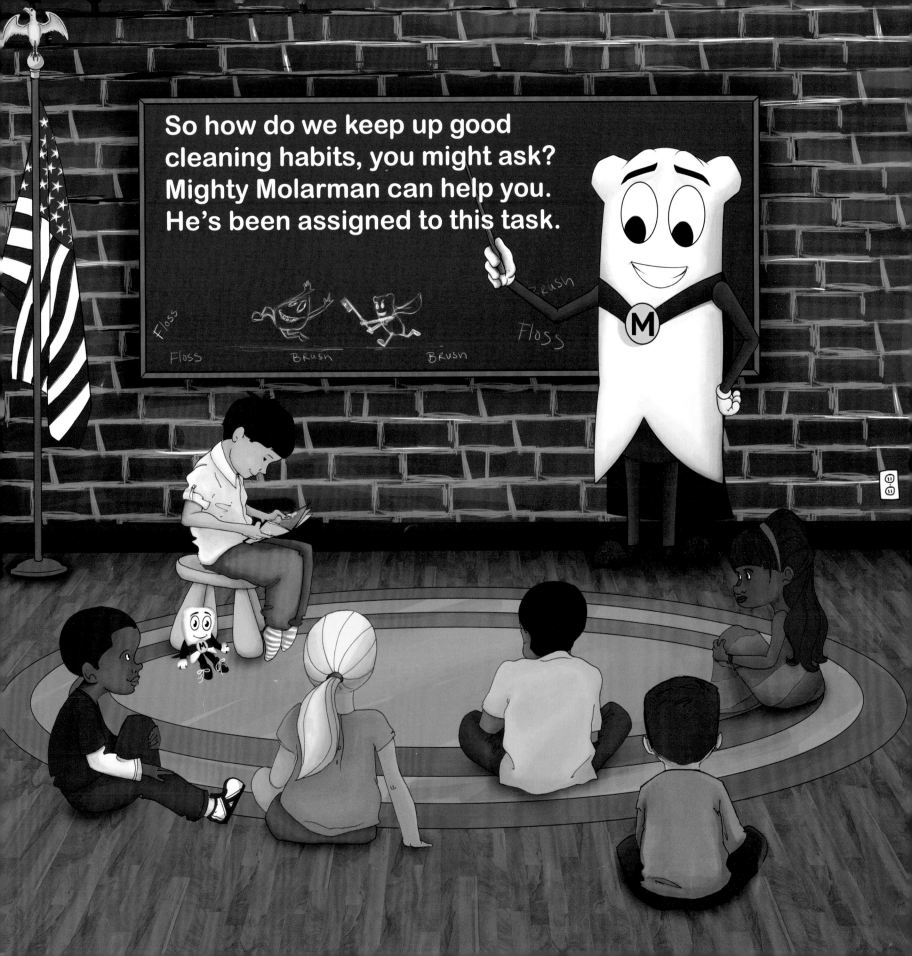

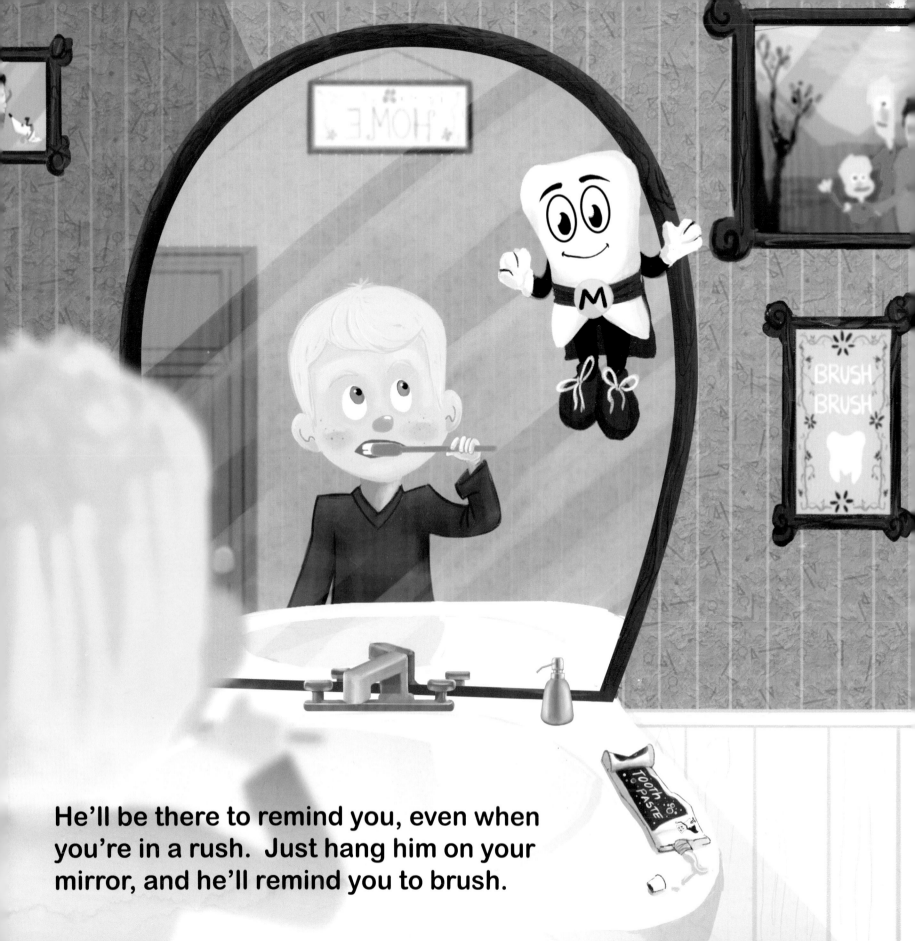

He'll be there to remind you, even when you're in a rush. Just hang him on your mirror, and he'll remind you to brush.

When you practice good dental hygiene, every single day, your smile will be healthy, and you'll keep Bacteria Boy away.

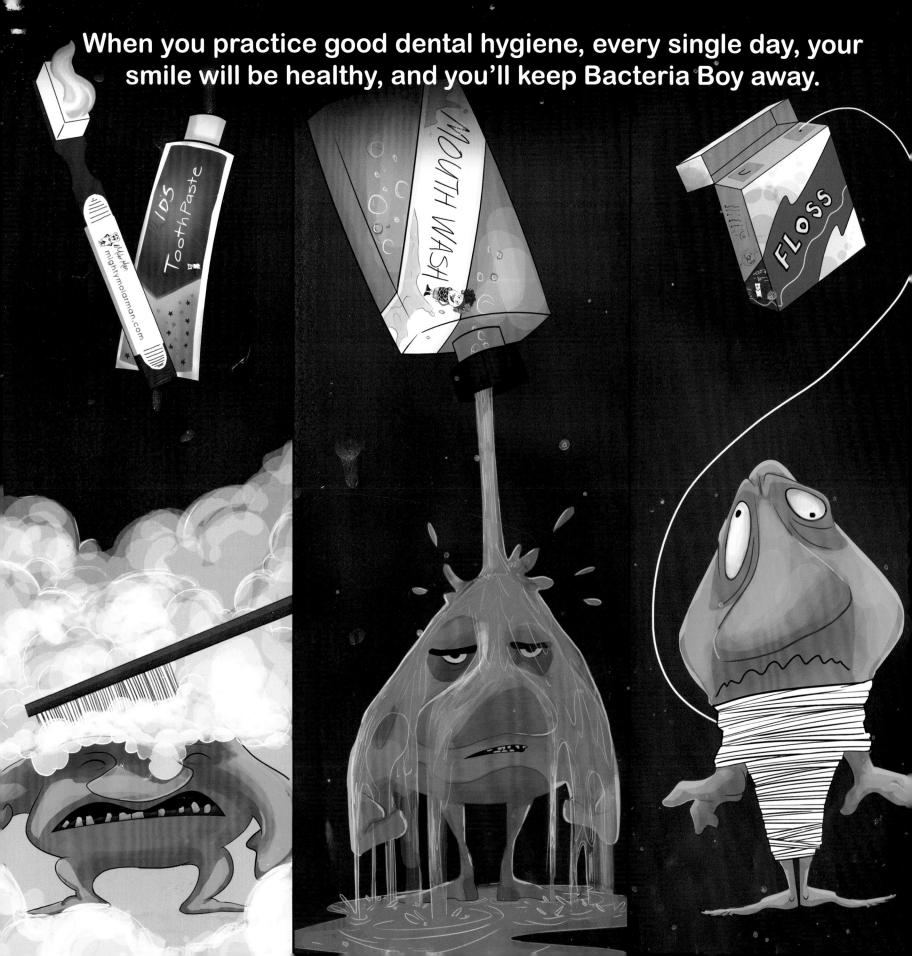

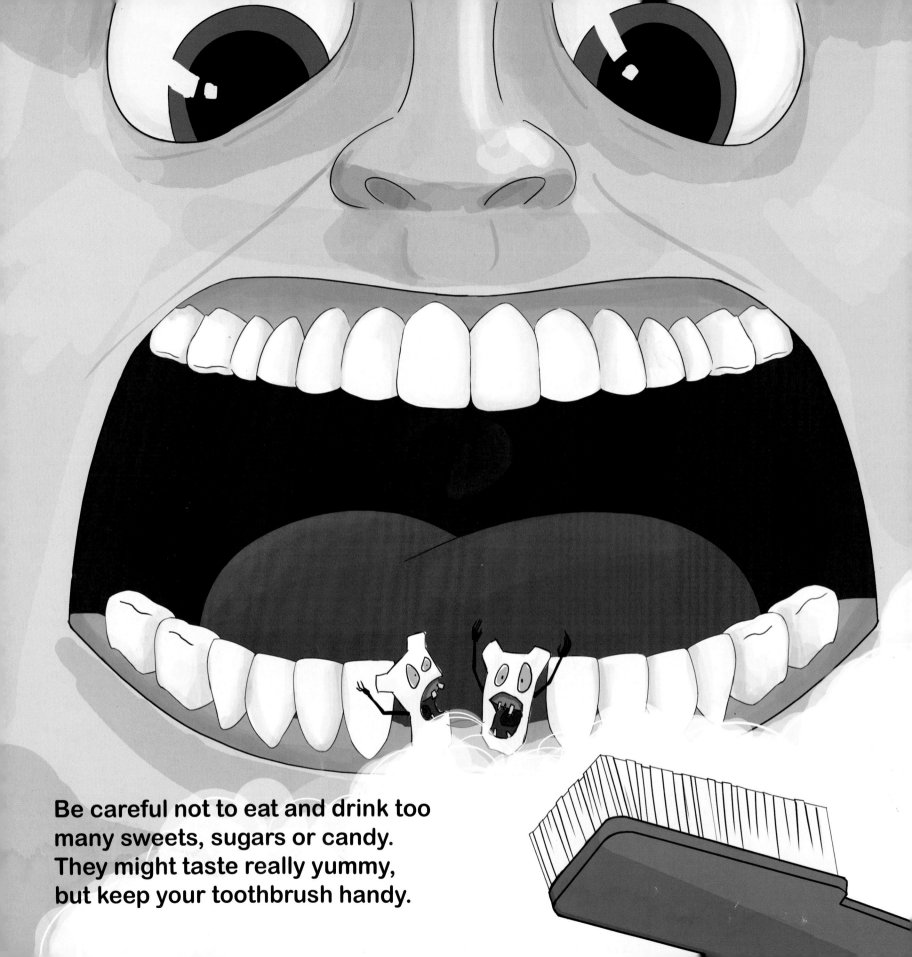

Be careful not to eat and drink too many sweets, sugars or candy. They might taste really yummy, but keep your toothbrush handy.

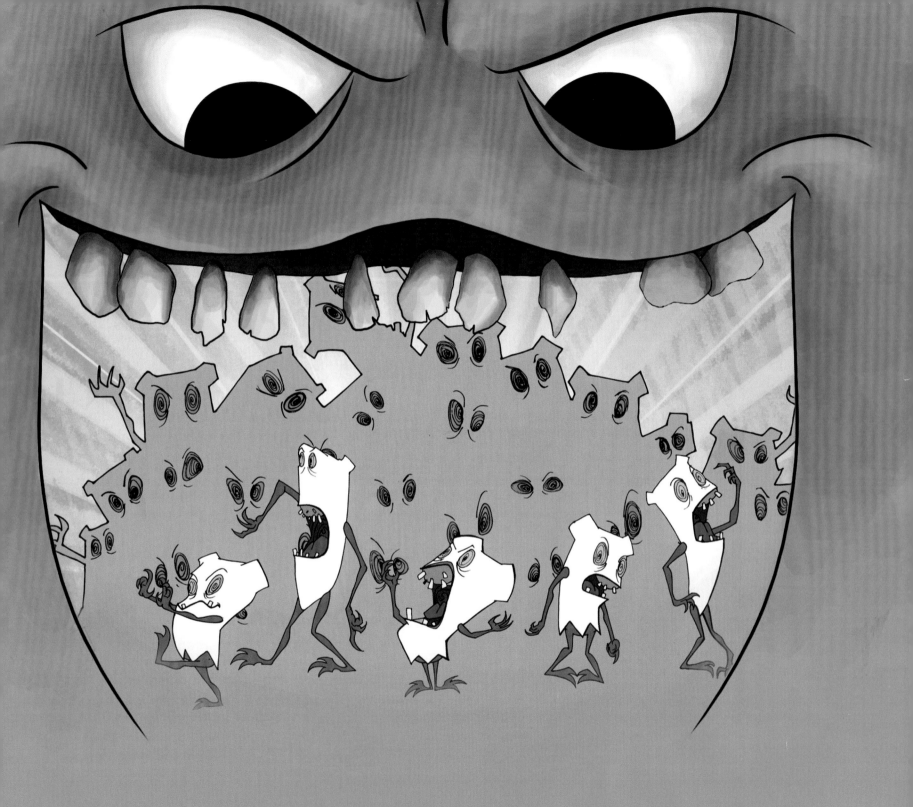

You see, Mighty Molarman's enemy is Bacteria Boy.
He causes lots of trouble; it's your smile he can destroy.

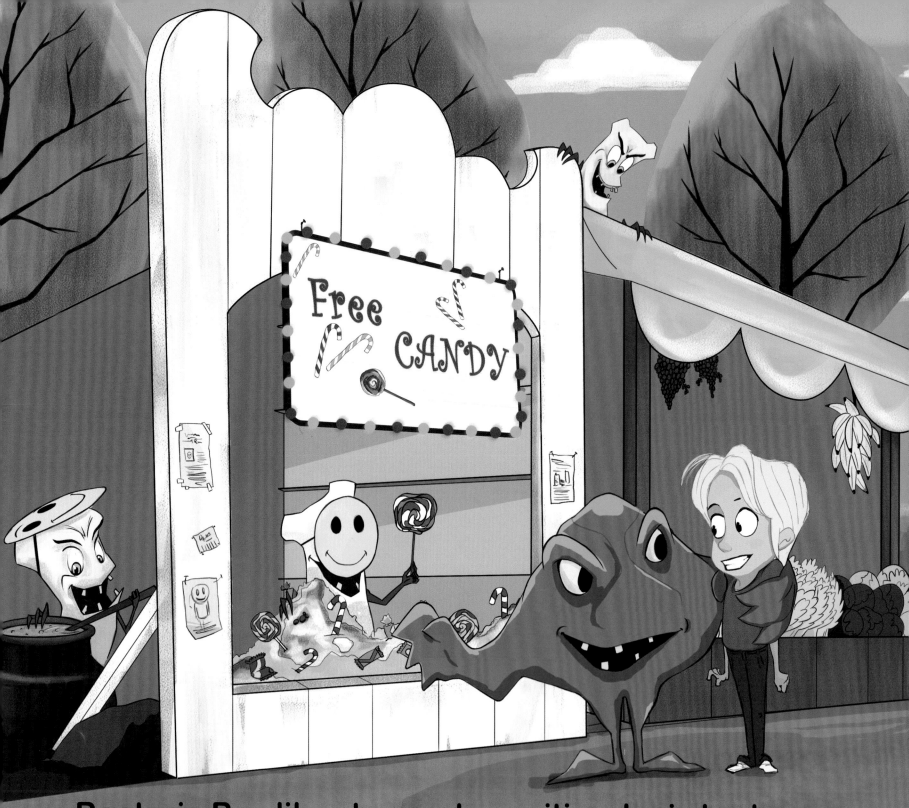

Bacteria Boy likes to create cavities, he is bad news.
He tempts children with sugary sweets,
when it's fruit and veggies you should choose.

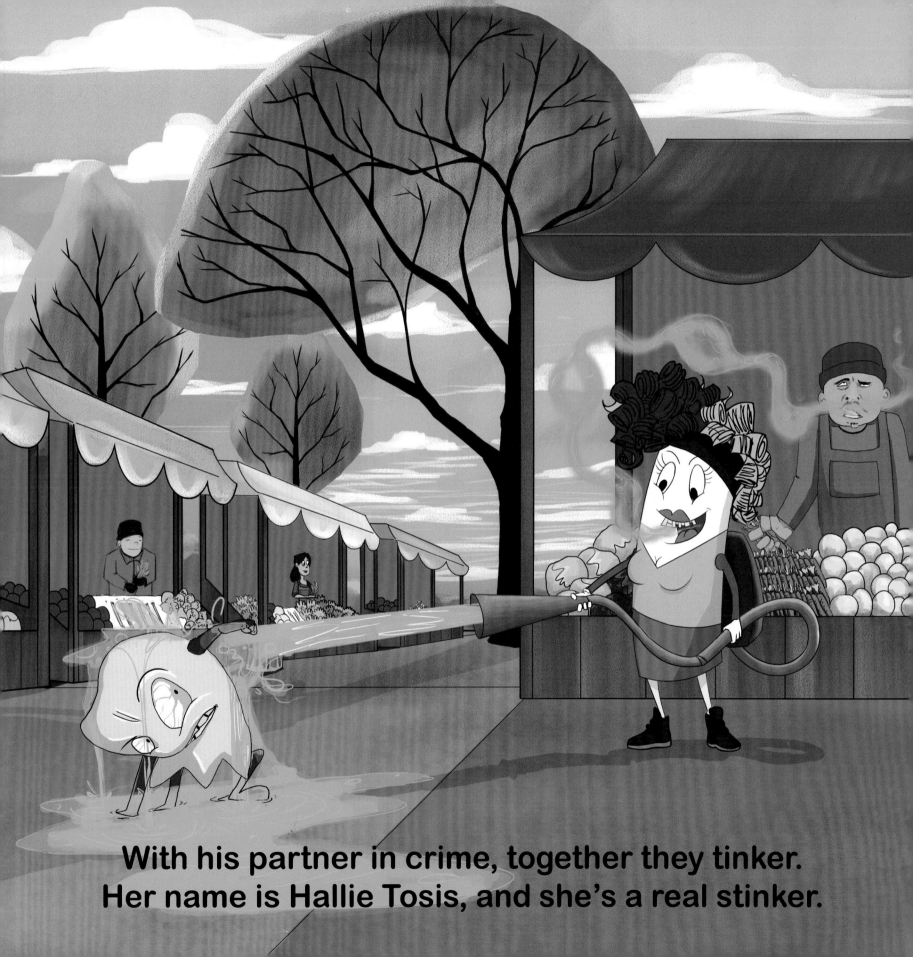

With his partner in crime, together they tinker.
Her name is Hallie Tosis, and she's a real stinker.

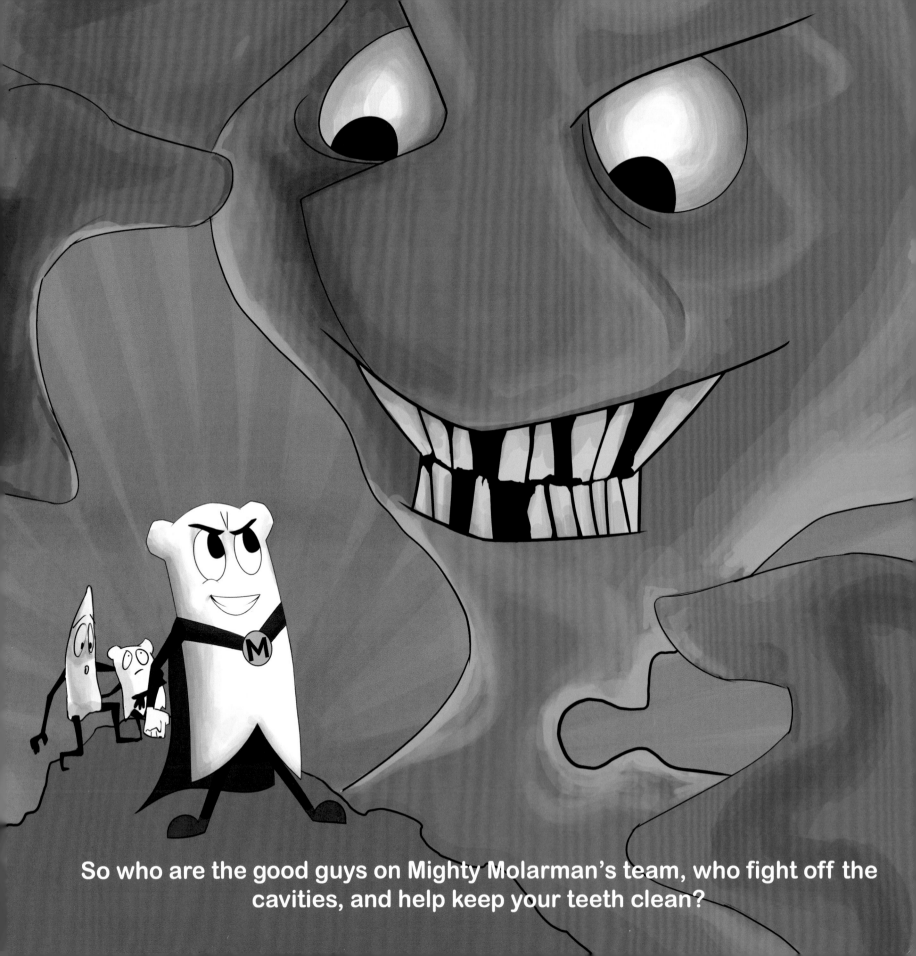

So who are the good guys on Mighty Molarman's team, who fight off the cavities, and help keep your teeth clean?

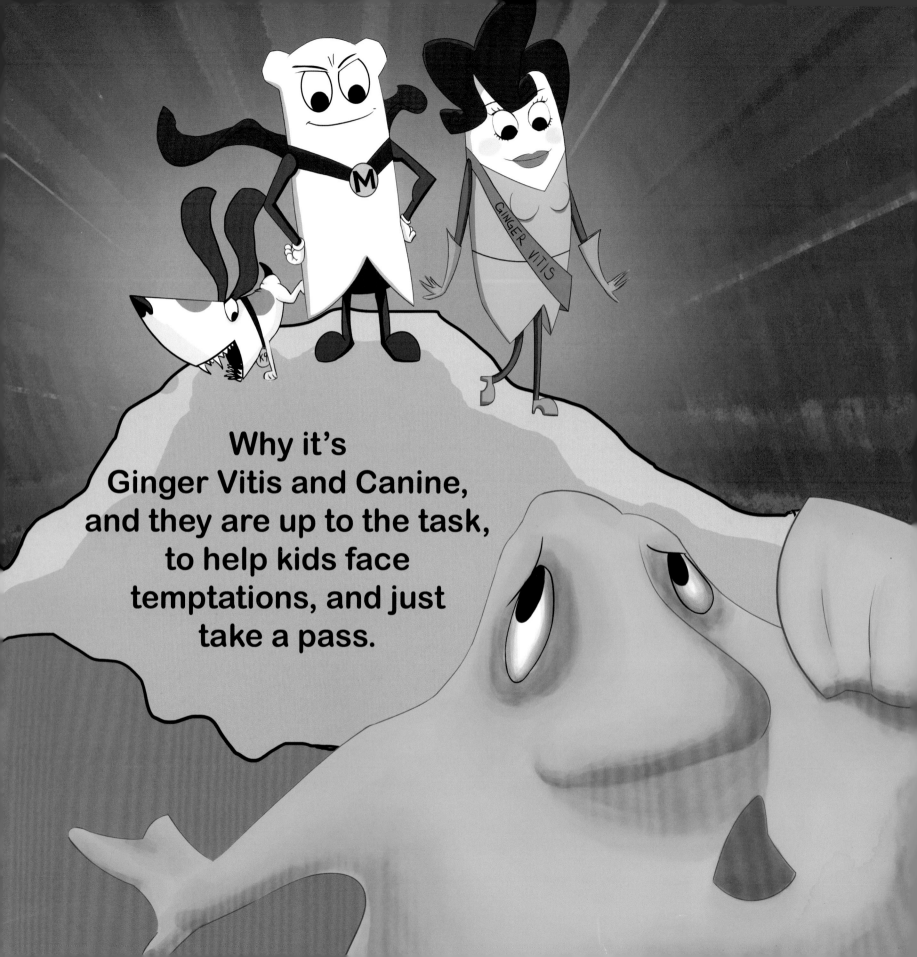

Why it's
Ginger Vitis and Canine,
and they are up to the task,
to help kids face
temptations, and just
take a pass.

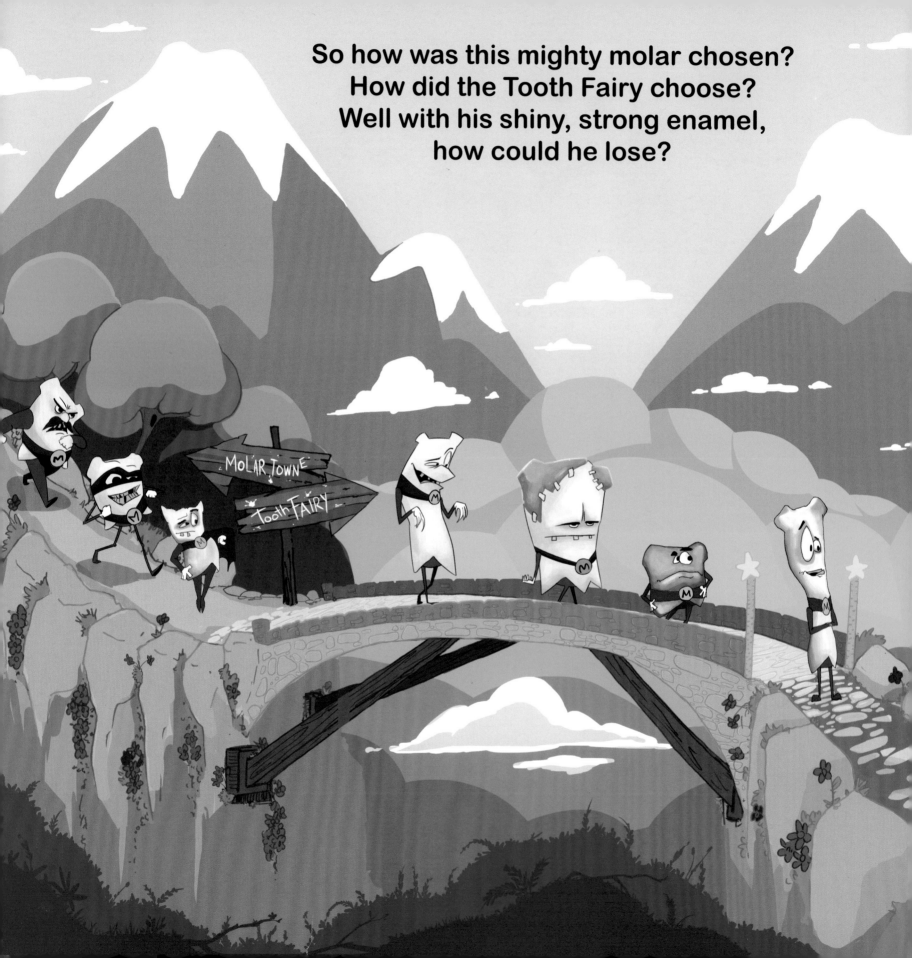

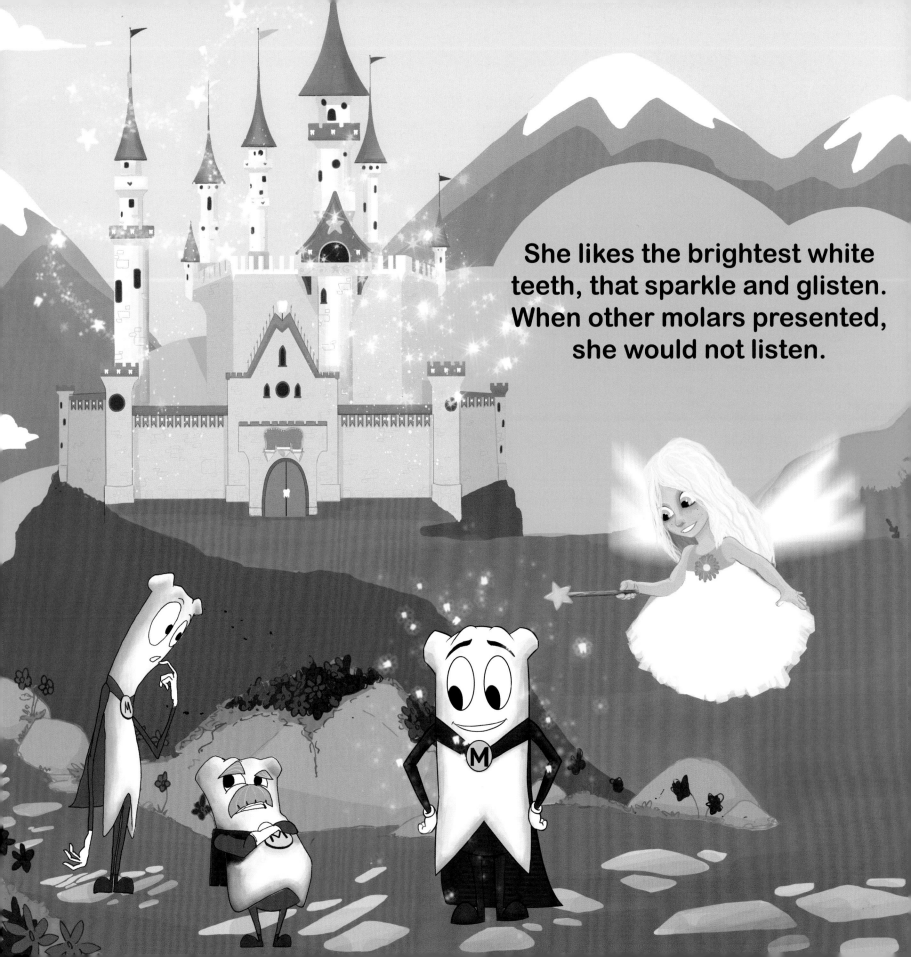

She likes the brightest white teeth, that sparkle and glisten. When other molars presented, she would not listen.

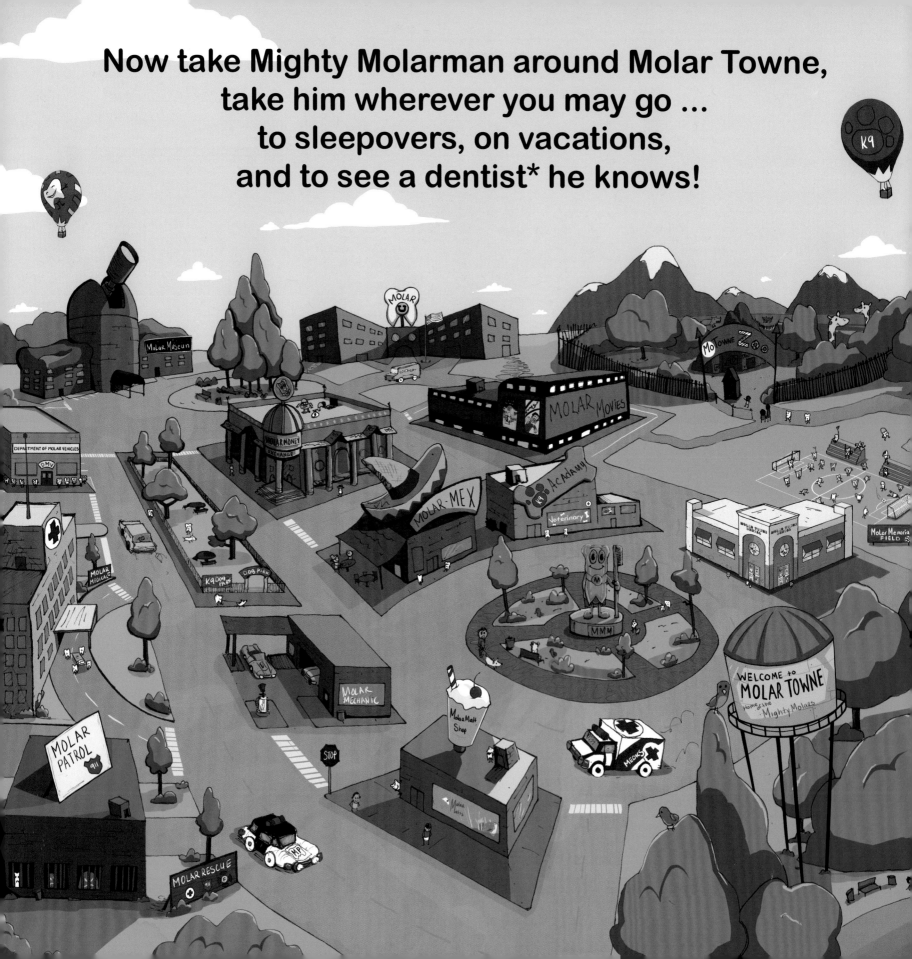

Now take Mighty Molarman around Molar Towne,
take him wherever you may go ...
to sleepovers, on vacations,
and to see a dentist* he knows!

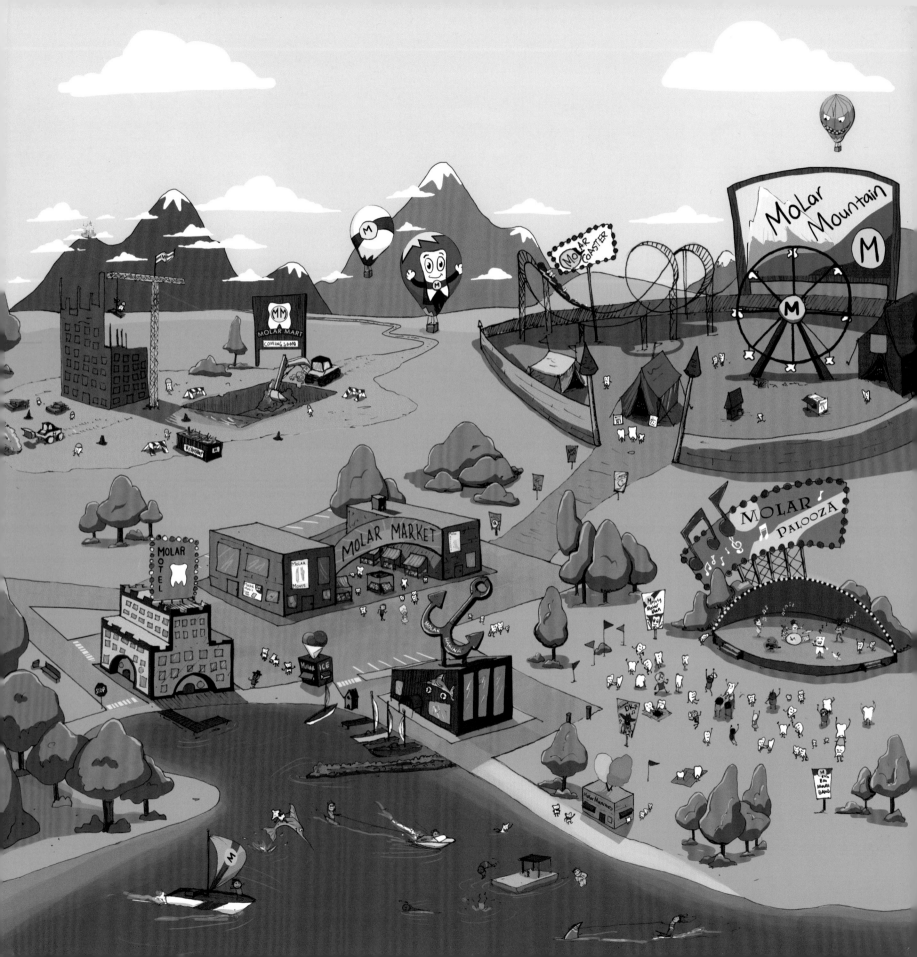

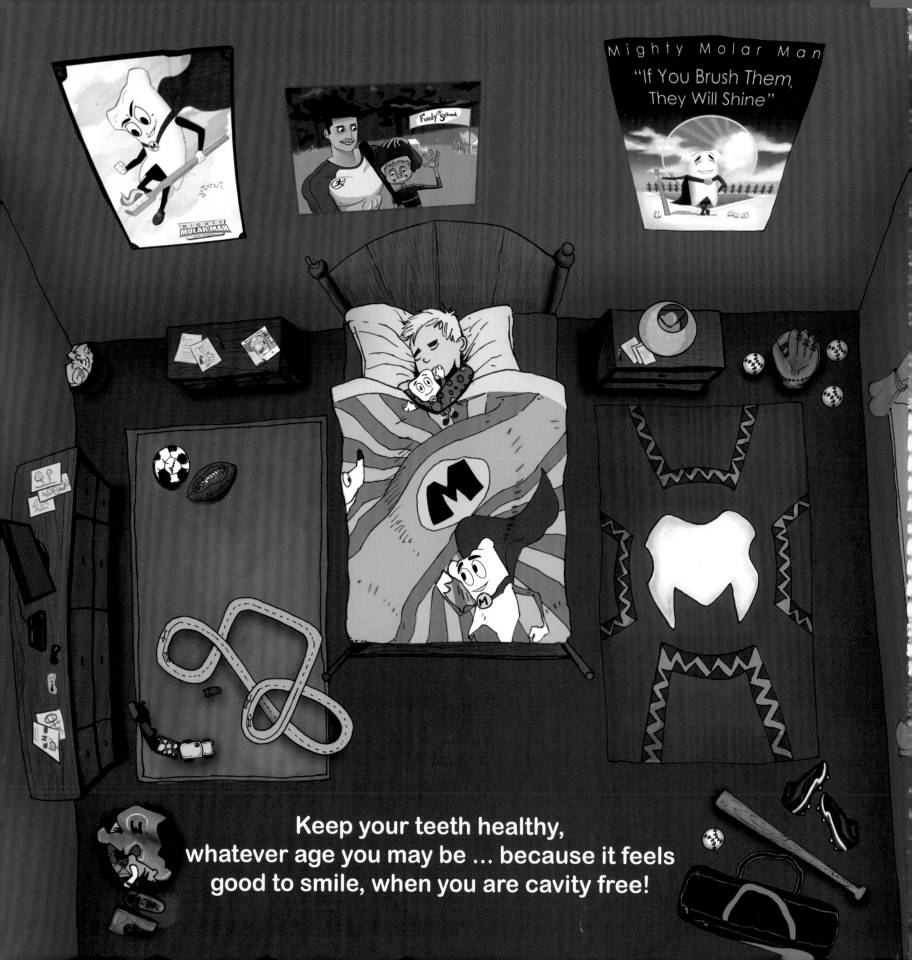

Keep your teeth healthy,
whatever age you may be ... because it feels
good to smile, when you are cavity free!

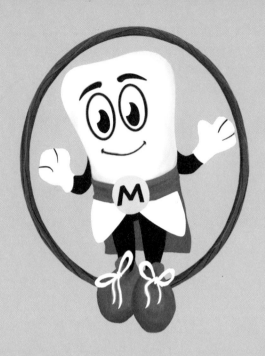

ISBN: 978-0-692-29215-0

Printed in Canada

mightymolarman.com

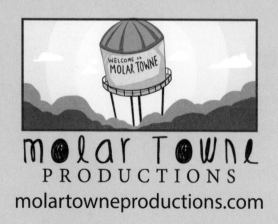

molartowneproductions.com